EASY
ALTERNATE DAY
FASTING

Fast and Feast Your Way
to a New You

by
Beth Christian

D0168031

Easy
Alternate Day
Fasting

Copyright © 2013
MadeGlobal Publishing

ISBN-13: 978-1482055016
ISBN: 1482055015

M
MadeGlobal Publishing

For more information on
MadeGlobal Publishing, visit our website
www.madeglobal.com

DISCLAIMER

The information and recipes provided in this book are designed to provide helpful information on Alternate Day Fasting. This book is not intended to be a substitute for consulting with your physician and any dietary change should be discussed with your physician, particularly if you have a medical condition. Neither the publisher nor the author shall be liable or responsible for any loss, damage or adverse reaction allegedly arising from the information or recipes given in this book.

While the author has made every effort to give accurate measurements, calorie counts, names of publications and website addresses, neither the author nor the publisher assumes any responsibility for errors or changes that occur after publication. The author and publisher also do not take any responsibility for third party books, websites and their content.

CONTENTS

INTRODUCTION

People are growing, and not in a good way! According to a 2012 report from the Centers for Disease Control and Prevention, more than a third of American adults were obese in 2009-2010. Yes, 35.7% of Americans over the age of twenty had a BMI of 30 or more and were therefore at risk of obesity-related conditions, such as heart disease, stroke, certain types of cancer and type 2 diabetes.

The National Heart, Lung and Blood Institute points out that obesity happens one pound at a time, you don't suddenly become obese overnight. Ignoring the mommy tummy, beer belly and the pounds you put on each year can lead to serious health problems, particularly if you have a family history of something like heart disease. Carrying excess weight increases your risk of:

- Diabetes
- Coronary heart disease and stroke
- Some types of cancer
- Respiratory problems
- Musculoskeletal disorders
- Infertility
- Memory problems, cognitive disorders and depression

But, if you're anything like me, you are more concerned about how you look and feel. You can't wear the clothes you want to, you don't feel sexy and you feel self-conscious about your appearance. Your relationship with food has become a love-hate one; you love to treat yourself to something yummy, but you hate the fat it causes around your middle or on your hips. Your bookshelves are full of diet books and you've tried every diet known to man or woman. You may even have resorted to diet pills or you may be considering surgery. Your battle with food and with the 'bulge' has taken over your life and it's a battle you're not winning. Sound familiar?

Since giving birth to my first child back in 1997, my weight has yo-yoed. I'd go on a diet for a few months, get back to my 'ideal weight' and then go back to 'normal' eating, and, of course, eventually to the original weight!

I tried everything – counting points, having red days and green days, doing detox diets, going vegan, eating foods which were low fat/high protein/low carb/low GI etc. - and everything worked, but only temporarily and it was all such hard work. Either I'd get sick of all the preparation, cost and hassle involved, and stop the diet, or I'd get to a weight I felt happy with and then go back to my old ways. Up, down, up, down, went my weight, along with my self-esteem. Nothing worked in the long term, they were just quick fixes and I just couldn't hack spending every day of my life counting points or calories. There was more to life than that.

As I contemplated another diet, being fourteen pounds (or perhaps a little more!) over what I should be, I happened to watch a TV program on 'fasting' and its health benefits. What I learned in that hour of TV has changed how I think about food, has changed my figure (for the better!) and will lower my risk of suffering from all those nasty diseases I mentioned earlier. What's more is that it's something I can cope with on an on-going basis, it is a life-change rather than a quick fix.

Note: Don't panic at the word 'fasting', it's not the usual type of fasting that I'm going to be talking about.

I'm not going to bore you silly with statistics, scary information on heart disease or any more fluff; I'm going to launch into the important stuff – what it is, why it's good and how you do it. I always skip the first few chapters of diet books to get to the nitty-gritty, so I'm not going to waste your time with those pointless chapters. You need some background, but not tens of pages.

Those of you who love reading the fine detail will find the links you need in "Further Reading" and on my website **www.EasyAlternateDayFasting.com** where you'll find lots of interesting things. I've also set up a Pinterest page **www.pinterest.com/easyalternate/** where I will add interesting articles, research material and recipes.

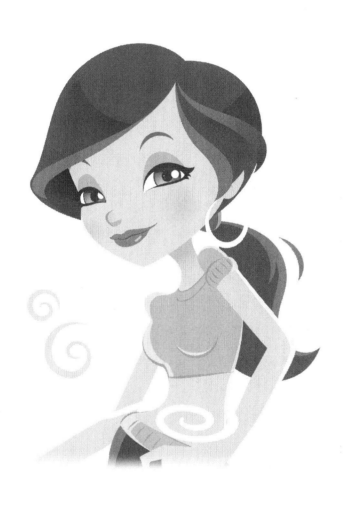

INITIAL CONSIDERATIONS

ARE YOU OVERWEIGHT?

We all know that being overweight is not good for us but what does "overweight" mean? How do you know if you're overweight or obese?

There are two types of calculations which can determine whether a person is overweight or carrying too much fat:

- **BMI (Body Mass Index)** – The idea of BMI is that it estimates how much body fat an individual is carrying based on their weight and height. It is calculated by dividing a person's mass by the square of their height. For adults, a healthy BMI is in the range of 18.5 to 24.9. You are overweight if you are between 25.0 and 30.0 and you are obese if your BMI is above 30.0. You will find an easy-to-use BMI calculator at: http://bit.ly/96tP2j

- **Waist Measurement** – Research has shown that carrying excess body fat in the abdominal area increases the risk of type 2 diabetes, cardiovascular disease and death, even when an individual has a healthy BMI. Your waist circumference (the measurement around your natural waist, just above the navel) should be less than 35 inches if you're a woman and less than 40 inches if you're a man.

If you have a BMI of over 24.9 and/or a waist circumference of 35 inches or over for a woman, or 40+ inches for a man, then you really need to lose some weight and body fat to get back to a healthy body.

WHY BOTHER LOSING WEIGHT?

It's easy to put off losing weight. You know there are risk factors involved in being overweight but you feel perfectly fine now so why bother? Well, there are many advantages to losing that fat:

- You'll have more energy
- You'll sleep better
- You'll feel sexier and be more confident
- You'll reduce your risk of all those nasty diseases and disorders already mentioned
- It'll be easier to take part in sports and activities
- Finding your size in clothes will be easier
- You might just be able to keep up with your kids or grandkids without being breathless or your joints aching
- You'll be able to wear those jeans, you know the ones that have been lurking at the back of your closet for the past 5+years because you always hoped that you'd be able to wear them again one day
- You'll get compliments
- It's an excuse to buy new clothes

Are you ready to change your life?

ALTERNATE DAY FASTING (ADF)

The word "fasting" might be a scary one. It makes us think of starvation and denial, and it's a bit of a turn-off really. Some fasting plans require people to abstain from food completely for a few days every month or two - just surviving on water, black tea or coffee, and perhaps miso soup – while others call for severe calorie restriction on a daily basis. Well, I don't know about you, but I couldn't handle either of those types of plans. I enjoy my food and I couldn't cope with the busy life I lead if I was fainting or couldn't concentrate. I'd also be highly likely to break the fast, I just don't have that much self-control!

Let me introduce you to Alternate Day Fasting, or ADF, which actually isn't fasting at all so don't worry. It's a kind of on-day/off-day diet and what is wonderful about it is that on the off-days (I call them Feast Days) you can eat and drink whatever you like, without the normal guilt you feel when you tuck into pizza, burger or, in my case, wine! You only have to be careful for half the week, or less if you want, and it's easy to follow – hurray!

Dr Krista Varady's Research

In the TV program I watched, BBC's "Horizon", journalist, physician and TV presenter Michael Mosley met Dr Krista Varady of the University of Illinois at Chicago. Dr Varady had just finished running a clinical trial, which is yet to be published, in which she put two groups of volunteers on a ten week ADF plan. On their fasting days, both groups were allowed one lunchtime meal of no more than 600 calories but their feed days (or Feast Days as I like to call them – yum!) were different. The first group were put on a low-fat diet on their Feast Days, while the second group were encouraged to eat a typical American diet, i.e. high fat.

Now, you'd expect both groups to lose weight because on alternate days they were of course only consuming 600 calories, when even on a typical low-calorie diet they'd be consuming 1500-2000 calories. But, you'd also expect those eating low-fat foods on their feed days to lose more weight, wouldn't you? Well, they didn't. Dr Varady found that those eating the typical high-fat diet on their feed days lost just as much weight and, in some cases, actually more than their low-fat counterparts. Both groups also benefited from falls in their blood pressure and LDL, or "bad", cholesterol. Good news!

Michael Mosley wanted to try out ADF but decided that he couldn't face doing it on alternate days. Instead, he did a 5:2 feed:fast plan, reducing his calorific intake to 600 calories on just two days a week and eating whatever he liked on the other five. He also decided to split the 600 calories into two meals: 300 calories for breakfast and 300 calories for an evening meal. After six weeks, he'd lost over fourteen pounds and had also changed his health for the better. Before he went on the 5:2 plan, he needed to take medication for high cholesterol and his blood glucose had been borderline diabetic. However, after just six weeks on the plan, both his cholesterol and blood glucose had gone down to the normal, healthy range. So happy with the results was Mosley, that he decided to carry on with the 5:2 plan indefinitely.

ADF AND *LEAN* *MASS* *PROTECTION*

What wasn't mentioned in the Horizon program was Dr Varady's research "Intermittent versus daily calorie restriction: which diet regimen is more effective for weight loss?" where she compared Alternate Day Fasting to diets which restricted calories on a daily basis, your standard low-calorie diet. Varady examined the effects of both types of 'diet' on weight loss, fat mass loss and lean mass (muscle) retention in people who were overweight or obese.

What Dr Varady found was that both groups of people lost weight, but the loss, in terms of fat loss and lean mass loss, was different. Those following a standard daily calorie restricted diet lost 75% of the weight as fat and 25% as fat free mass, whereas those following an intermittent calorie restriction plan lost 90% of the weight as fat and only 10% as fat free mass. These results suggest that intermittent calorie restriction plans, such as ADF or 5:2, are more effective at getting rid of body fat while also protecting lean mass. What was even more interesting was that the results were the same even if the individual on the standard daily calorie restricted diet was on a high protein diet. Dr Varady's research is still ongoing but these results are very encouraging, after all, it's fat that we want to lose!

THE BENEFITS OF ADF OR 5:2

According to Dr Varady's research, following an intermittent calories restriction plan, whether doing it on alternate days or 5:2. will give you the following benefits:

- Loss of body fat
- Retention of lean mass
- Decreased risk of obesity-related disorders, and those related to high cholesterol, high body fat, high blood pressure and high glucose levels.

Research carried out by other scientists looking at the effects of fasting on mice has also suggested that such eating plans may have anti-aging benefits. Mice who follow a calorie restricted diet live up to forty times longer than mice eating a normal diet and it appears that intermittent fasting, like ADF and 5:2, offers the same benefits as continuous calories restriction. This area requires further research, but intermittent fasting seems to slow the rate of cell turnover thus slowing down the aging process. I, for one, have found that my energy levels are increased and that I feel better in myself, so perhaps I will live to a grand old age!

MY EXPERIENCE OF ALTERNATE DAY FASTING

After watching the Horizon program and digging into the research behind ADF, I decided to give it a go. I had nothing to lose - well, actually I had a fair bit of weight to lose – and it sounded like the diet would be easy to follow and wouldn't cost me anything in fancy food and gadgets. So impressed was my husband with Dr Varady's research and Michael Mosley's results that he decided to join me on the plan.

We decided:

- To follow the ADF plan – one day would be calorie restricted, the next day would be completely normal, and so on...
- Fast Days would consist of a 400-600 calorie lunch any time between the hours of midday and 2pm. Our meals tend to be around 450-500 calories but we don't worry if we consume slightly more or less.
- On Fast Days drinks had to be water, black coffee/tea, herbal tea or zero calorie soft drinks.
- Feast Days would be completely unlimited and guilt-free.
- To weigh ourselves once a week.
- To be flexible if an event came up on a scheduled Fast Day – If that meant having two Feast days one after

another then we wouldn't feel guilty, we'd simply have the next day as a Fast Day.

I already had plenty of recipe books with low calorie meal ideas in so we used those and when we had to go out for the day or we couldn't be bothered to do a recipe then we made use of meal replacement shakes and bars. We were pleasantly surprised by how easy it was to do.

At the start, we noticed that we both got quite irritable on Fast Days and we found that it was best to plan the Fast Day meal the day before (on the Feast Day) so that we knew what we were having, how many calories it had in it and could go food shopping if needed. It's really not much fun doing food shopping on a Fast Day, believe me!

THE RESULTS

After three months of following the ADF plan my husband and I noticed that we had:

- Raised energy levels.
- Less of an appetite on Feast Days – I thought I'd want to eat anything and everything, but I found myself saying 'no' to things, eating smaller portions and leaving food on my plate.
- Less hunger on Fast Days – The first few fast days were hard, but it soon became part of my routine and I certainly didn't feel ravenous all the time. I once read that it takes six weeks for something to become a habit and then it becomes automatic. This is definitely the case with an eating plan like ADF.
- Lost a steady 2lbs per week on average
- Lost fat – Unfortunately, neither of us thought to measure our waists, hips, bottoms, arms etc. before we

started but both of us moved several holes on our jeans belts and I can wear skirts and trousers that I haven't worn in quite a long time. My new party trick is pulling my jeans down without unzipping or unbuttoning them! My extra chin also disappeared! We bought a new bathroom scale with built-in fat monitor and our body fat percentages steadily decreased too.

- Returned to a healthy weight – To be in your forties and to be the weight you were in your early 20s, when you were at your fittest, really is a wonderful feeling.
- Stuck to a plan! - I have never ever stuck to a "diet" for more than a few weeks so this was a first. I'm one of those people who finds it hard to stick to rules so when something is banned in a diet I just feel the need to eat it and then I fall off the wagon and give up. With ADF, I knew that I only had to be "good" for 24 hours so I could wait.

NOW IT IS YOUR TURN...

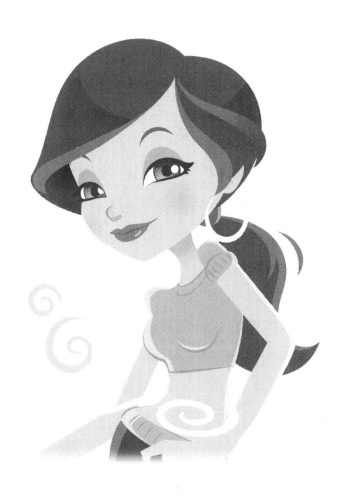

ADF and 5:2 Plan Instructions

What's great about Alternate Day Fasting and the 5:2 plan, is that they're both easy to follow and Dr Varady's research has shown that people find them easier to stick to. Calorie counting on alternate days (or just twice a week for 5:2) is so much easier than doing it all of the time. You're also not tempted to be 'naughty' on Fast Days because you know that you can be as 'naughty' as you like the next day. No food is banned, so you don't have that sense of denial or the worry that you'll fail. How many times have you started a diet and then given up because you've fallen off the wagon? With ADF or 5:2 you simply live for today.

The Basics

I'm not going to give you pages and pages of instructions and guidance. What a waste of time when I can just tell you:

Fast Day = Maximum of 600 calories

Feast Day = Eat what you like

For Alternate Day Fasting, simply fast one day and feast the next.

For the 5:2 plan, simply feast on five days and fast on two. Split up your two days, though. DO NOT fast on two consecutive days because that would be pure hell!

That's it. Easy peasy!

If you like, you can split your calories into two meals, like Michael Mosley did, but I found it easier to have one main meal and to aim for 500 calories as my total. I have my meal at lunchtime. I don't snack and I'm not tempted to, I just make sure that I have plenty of fluids and having a drink when you feel hunger pangs really does help.

I'm sure most of you won't be phased by the idea of making a meal that adds up to 400-600 calories because you'll have as many diet cookbooks as I have. However, if you've never counted a calorie in your life (lucky you!) then you may need some guidance. Fortunately, we live in an enlightened world and you'll find calorie counts on food labels or, in the case of things like fresh fruit and vegetables, online on calorie counters and in food databases. I have also produced a book of 100 recipes to help you – see "100 Under 500 Calorie Meals" by Beth Christian.

CALCULATING CALORIES

If you're not following a recipe which has the calories already counted, then you will want to know how to calculate the calories in the food you're eating.

I'm not going to bore you with the whole scientific bit about what calories are - they're a unit of energy – because that doesn't help you count them. What you need to know is that you're going to be looking for the words "calories" or "kilo calories" or "kcal" on food packaging. Don't use "kilojoules" or "kj", they're not the right thing.

Food packaging tends to have the nutritional information split into "per serving" (and it gives the weight for a standard serving) and "per 100g". You may need to get your calculator out if you're not having a standard serving or 100g of that food. So, what do you do? Well, if a serving of a particular food is 224g and that serving has 180 calories, you'll want to know how many calories there are in 1g.

180 calories divided by 224g = 0.80

1g = 0.8 calories

If you're going to be using 100g of that food, then you will be consuming 80 calories (100g x 0.8 calories = 80 calories).

For something like an apple, you can use an online calorie counter or database such as http://bit.ly/Vb6Fbc

If you type in "apple" on that website, it comes up with "Apples, raw, with skin" and then you can choose your serving size to calculate the calories.

If you're eating out, you can either do it the easy way and change that day to a Feast Day, or you can go somewhere where the menu is calorie counted or they have nutritional information online. Burger King and McDonald's, for example, both have nutritional information for their menus online:

http://bit.ly/skY19 for Burger King
http://bit.ly/okO8b3 for McDonalds

Using Recipes

I've included twenty recipes in this e-book for main meals. All these recipes are delicious and are 500 calories or less, so you can also add something like a low-calorie yogurt or cereal bar. You can also use your favorite diet recipes or have a look on my website:

www.EasyAlternateDayFasting.com

Also read my recipe book for inspiration:

"100 Under 500 Calorie Meals" by Beth Christian

If you want to keep things simple, grilled fish or chicken with steamed vegetables make for a delicious and low calorie meal, and you can add a low-calorie dessert to finish it off. For a picnic, we've enjoyed ham or tuna salad wraps plus a low-calorie cereal bar.

Make a list of your favorite recipes, noting down the calorie count, so you can enjoy them again.

Hidden Naughties and Bad Habits

On Fast Days, you will need to account for every single thing you consume, food and drink. If you butter your bread, add ketchup to your meal or mayo to your sandwich, then you must count those calories too. Also don't forget to account for drinks.

One thing I used to find hard on Fast Days, but which has got easier over time, is preparing food for my children. Who doesn't help themselves to a fry or two as they serve up? Well, I don't now! Sometimes, people don't even realise that they're doing it, so just be aware of habits like that.

DIETING TIPS

Be flexible – If a Fast Day doesn't fit in with your schedule then change it. If something suddenly comes up and your Fast Day turns into a Feast Day then don't worry, simply fast the next day. Don't beat yourself up, there's no failing with this plan.

Plan your Fast Day meal on a Feast Day – It's easier to calculate calories on a full stomach.

Don't go food shopping on Fast Days – it's cruel.

Keep hydrated – Water is the best drink, but we also enjoy green tea and herbal teas.

Get a drink (zero calorie) when you feel hungry – Thirst is often confused with hunger anyway.

Vary your diet – Meal replacement bars and shakes are convenient, but can get boring. Try out new recipes and new ways of preparing food. My husband often comments that we eat better now because we try new and tasty meals.

Keep active – Exercise is good for you, we all know that!

Make a note of favourite recipes – this way you can have those meals again easily.

Have a "fall back" plan – I eat an egg sandwich (made with low fat mayo) and two cereal bars when I'm in a hurry on a fast day. I know the calorie count of this meal by heart so I don't have to work anything out.

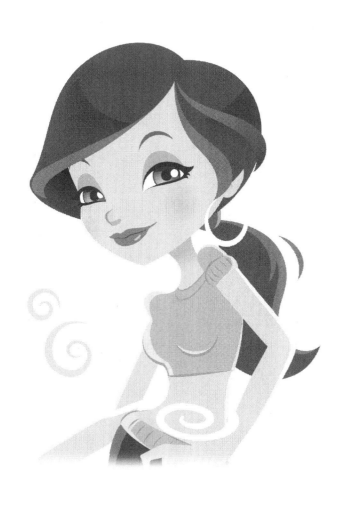

Why ADF is Better than Other Diets or Programs

I'm a diet veteran and this is the only plan that's worked for me. Here are some reasons why:

- Nothing is banned
- You don't have to hunt high and low for special foods or supplements that nobody has heard of
- It's easy to follow
- It's flexible and fits into anyone's life
- You don't have to cook separate meals for yourself all the time
- You live for today
- You see results and they are ongoing
- It's nice to know that if you're feeling hungry and deprived today that you can eat as much as you like tomorrow
- When someone asks you out for a meal you can go and enjoy yourself without feeling guilty
- Thanksgiving, Christmas, Birthdays etc. can be enjoyed without the usual guilt
- The candy bar that's calling out to you today can be enjoyed tomorrow, rather than in six months' time
- It's not a temporary plan that you then finish, go back to normal and put on weight, it's a life change

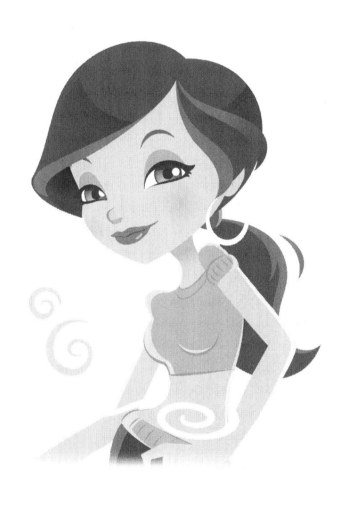

Your Maintenance Plan

Once you're at your ideal weight you're going to want to stay that way and it's easy with ADF, you just need to find the balance of fasting and feasting which works for you.

I was fasting on alternate days when I was losing weight so to maintain my healthy weight I changed to the 5:2 plan, i.e. fasting for two days each week. That worked for me but my husband found that he carried on losing weight doing 5:2 so he fasts for just one day a week now. Experiment and see what works for you.

What's great about the Fasting/Feasting approach when you're in the "maintenance" phase is that if you go on vacation and put on a few pounds then you can simply increase the number of fast days when you get back until you reach your goal weight again. It is flexible and you're in control.

The plan is a long-term life change, rather than a diet. I've been fasting and feasting for six months now and this is the first time that I have ever felt completely in control of my weight and my health. I don't panic about meals out, all-you-can-eat buffets and vacations, and I don't feel guilty about eating "bad" food any more; I am in control of my weight for the first time ever – phew!

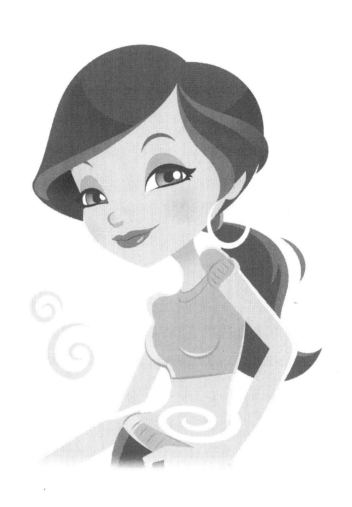

FAQs

WILL I FEEL HUNGRY?

Yes. There's no way round it. You're used to eating what you like when you like and suddenly you'll be cutting down to 500 calories on alternate days, so you're bound to feel hungry. What's good about it is that you'll learn to recognise hunger. Too often we mistake thirst for hunger so try having a glass of water or zero calorie drink.

You'll soon get used to the 'regime' and the hunger won't bother you because you'll know that the next day you can completely pig out if you want to.

HOW MUCH WEIGHT WILL I LOSE?

Different people lose at different rates so it's impossible to say. My husband lost more each week than I did. He lost 2-3 pounds whereas I tended to lose 1-2 pounds. You'll probably find that you'll lose more at the beginning of the diet and then it will become steady.

How do I maintain my weight when I've reached my goal?

You'll need to experiment. Try doing two days a week (not consecutive days) as fast days and the other five as feast days and if you still lose weight then just do one day a week as a fast day. Intermittent fasting is good for your health so do make fasting a regular thing as you'll only put all the weight back on if you go back to your old ways.

What do I do when I go on vacation?

Don't worry about fasting when you're on vacation, just enjoy yourself. You can get back to normal when you return.

How do I find the calorie count of foods?

Packaged foods tend to have nutritional information on them so you need to look for calories per serving (or kcal) or per 100g and then weigh out how much you're going to consume. There are also online calorie counters which give the calories in branded foods or foods like a standard medium egg or an apple. It really is easy to find the calorific value of foods these days.

What can I eat? Help!

On feast days you can eat whatever you like and on fast days you are allowed a maximum of 500 calories. See our example 2 week plan and recipes for some inspiration or get a copy of our recipe book. Alternatively, you can simply count calories by using food labels.

I have stand-by meals for those days where I'm too busy to count calories or worry about food. For example, I know that an egg mayo sandwich, cup of soup and two cereal bars add up to under 500 calories but also fill me and keep me going so that's what I have when I have no inspiration and haven't got time to cook.

How do I handle eating out?

Be flexible and change your routine so that your meal out happens on a feast day. If something comes up out of the blue then don't worry about it, enjoy your meal and then have a fast day the next day.

What do I do if I eat more than 500 calories on a fast day?

Don't panic! It's not the end of the world. Tomorrow is another day and you can turn the day into a feast day and fast the next day. Problem solved!

Help! My fast day turned into a feast day! What do I do?

Fast tomorrow and don't feel guilty. This plan is meant to be flexible so don't beat yourself up about it.

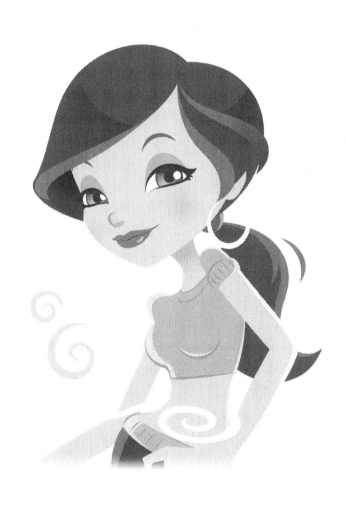

Your First 2 Weeks

The suggested recipes on the next page are included in this book's recipe section at the back of the book, along with some other delicious calorie counted meals. If you want to substitute another 500 calorie meal, that is fine and won't affect the diet at all. If you are looking for a wide selection of suitable recipes then why not check out the book "100 Under 500 Calorie Meals" (by me, Beth Christian) and see what interests you!

Remember this one simple step:

FEAST DAY   Eat and drink as much as you like of anything you like

FAST DAY   One mail meal of 500 calories maximum, drinks must be calorie free (water is best!)

WEEK ONE

DAY	FAST/FEAST	SUGGESTED RECIPE
Monday	FEAST	Your choice!
Tuesday	FAST	Curried Chicken Kebabs with brown rice and salad (480 calories in total)
Wednesday	FEAST	-
Thursday	FAST	Chicken in Mushroom Sauce with egg noodles, string beans and an apple (488 calories in total)
Friday	FEAST	-
Saturday	FAST	Baked Shellfish Paella (292 calories) and an Apple Crumb Pie (168 calories)
Sunday	FEAST	-

WEEK TWO

DAY	FAST/FEAST	SUGGESTED RECIPE
Monday	FAST	Swordfish Steak with Yogurt Parsley Sauce, assorted grilled vegetables and a wholegrain roll (455 calories in total)
Tuesday	FEAST	-
Wednesday	FAST	Crispy Oven Fried Chicken served with duck sauce for dipping, spinach and sweet potato (478 calories in total)
Thursday	FEAST	-
Friday	FAST	Boneless Pork Provence Style served with boiled potatoes, apple for dessert (total of 475 calories)
Saturday	FEAST	-
Sunday	FAST	Curried Vegetarian Stew served with rice and plain yogurt (495 calories in total)

CONCLUSION

The Easy Alternate Day Fasting diet is a truly amazing way to lose weight and regain the healthy body you once had. I say this as Beth's husband, and also as someone who has followed the diet plan within this book. It really works.

My experience of the plan has been really profound, so I hope you don't mind me sharing it with you.

Now, I can't say that I was overweight before starting the diet, in fact I exercise regularly, lead an active lifestyle and I *thought* that I ate reasonably healthily. None the less, I am approaching my 40th birthday and the weight had started to go on around my middle. I wasn't as trim as I wanted to be.

I'm honestly not someone who ever thought about going on a diet. Quite the opposite in fact. I was happy to watch Beth try out the latest thing in diets and enjoy the positive results. But I did not like the aftermath of it all: Beth's frustration when the results did not last long or did not work as well as she had hoped, and it has to be said that some of the diets were pretty strange too!

When I heard about the possible health benefits of The Alternate Day Diet, it was something that I wanted to try along with Beth, as it meant we could eat our normal food on "feast" days, and limiting calories on "fast" days turned out to be just fine. I couldn't believe how quickly the changes in my own body happened. It was really incredible to see.

Would you believe that I first felt the difference in my fingers. Strange but true! With the rest of your clothes you can tighten your belt without knowing it and you don't immediately notice that your shirt and top are looser. But on my fingers I noticed that my wedding ring felt a little more loose on my finger. This was after only a few weeks of fasting and feasting. It opened my eyes that this diet really was working. Fast forward ten weeks and my belt was on the tightest hole and some of the jeans that I had bought over the last few years were what I would now call too big. It was a fantastic feeling. I look in the mirror and think "Looking GOOD!".

After 12 weeks, I was down to the weight that I was when I used to be at university. That is, the same weight I was when I was 19 years old and in to rock climbing and weight lifting. Not only that, the weight lost had been easily controlled and from all the right places - my stomach looks great now! It was a loss of fat, not of muscle.

Yes, during the early stages of the diet I did feel hungry on fast days. Beth had told me that it would be a little tricky. But it wasn't too bad, and quite honestly it makes you appreciate the food you do eat a lot more! It is a good thing, and the quick and sustained results speak for themselves. Even friends who I don't see very often comment on my weight loss and how healthy I look. I didn't even think I was overweight!

I'll just share one more aspect of the Easy Alternate Day Fasting plan. As the diet went on, I noticed my body fat percentage dropping. Early on, we invested in a digital bathroom scale which could measure the percentage of fat in your body, and it kept on going down and down. I am now exactly where I want to be in weight, in looks and most importantly in body fat levels. I know that my body will last much longer in this state, that my knees won't wear out, that I'm now very unlikely to have a heart attack or to get diabetes. With much more energy, a healthier body and a much lower fat percentage, I am a happy person! I'm well and truly established in the "maintenance" part of the diet and will be sticking with it for life. I'm not giving up my new look for anything!

A final thought to leave you with - Beth is also looking more stunning now than she has ever done. This diet has worked the same wonders in her that it has done in me. I'm so glad that we both started Alternate Day Fasting together.

I know that you'll have just as much success in creating the healthy lifestyle you want, getting the body you have dreamed of and generally improving your health if you follow the Easy Alternate Day Fasting method.

To your success and health!

Pete Christian
(Husband of Beth Christian)

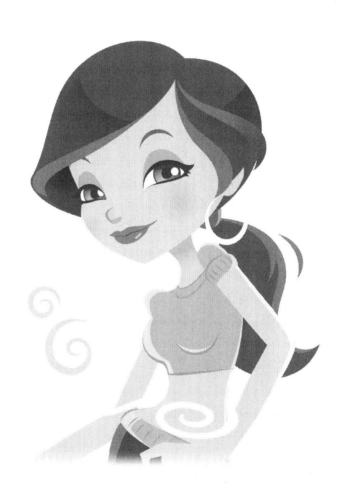

FURTHER READING

- Intermittent versus daily calorie restriction: which diet regimen is more effective for weight loss? K. A. Varady of Department of Kinesiology and Nutrition, University of Illinois at Chicago - bit.ly/13HASiz
- The 5:2 diet: can it help you lose weight and live longer? Michael Mosley - bit.ly/QGqQoL
- Improvements in Coronary Heart Disease Risk Indicators by Alternate-Day Fasting Involve Adipose Tissue Modulations, Surabhi Bhutani, Monica C. Klempel, Reed A. Berger and Krista A. Varady - bit.ly/YbpFaq
- Intermittent fasting dissociates beneficial effects of dietary restriction on glucose metabolism and neuronal resistance to injury from calorie intake, R. Michael Anson, Zhihong Guo, Rafael de Cabo, Titilola Iyun, Michelle Rios, Adrienne Hagepanos, Donald K. Ingram, Mark A. Lane, and Mark P. Mattson - bit.ly/IyxJps
- Intermittent Food Deprivation Improves Cardiovascular and Neuroendocrine Responses to Stress in Rats, Ruiqian Wan, Simonetta Camandola, and Mark P. Mattson - bit.ly/13HBEfj
- The effect on health of alternate day calorie restriction: Eating less and more than needed on alternate days prolongs life, James B. Johnson, Donald R. Laub, Sujit John - bit.ly/VCE5x6

- Fasting every other day, while cutting few calories, may reduce cancer risk, Sarah Yang - bit.ly/7JAHf3
- Apparent Prolongation of the Life Span of Rats by Intermittent Fasting, Anton J. Carlson and Frederick Hoelzel - bit.ly/UwqJkz
- How fasting could help you slow down the ageing process, Roger Dobson, Daily Mail - bit.ly/cZf0[a]n
- Alternate-day fasting and chronic disease prevention: a review of human and animal trials, K A Varady and M K Hellerstein - 1.usa.gov/VCEbVC
- Researcher: Fasting preserves brain as well as body - bit.ly/KSiB7Q
- Time-Restricted Feeding without Reducing Caloric Intake Prevents Metabolic Diseases in Mice Fed a High-Fat Diet, M Hatori et al. - 1.usa.gov/LhnHwB

RECIPES

CURRIED CHICKEN KEBABS

Aromatic skewers of tender and flavorful chicken and vegetables hit the grill for a quick and healthy dinner.

INGREDIENTS

- 1 tbsp. curry powder
- 1 tbsp. nonfat plain yogurt
- Juice of 1 lemon
- 1 tbsp. agave nectar or honey
- 8 oz. boneless skinless chicken breasts, cubed
- 1 medium bell pepper, seeded and cut into chunks
- 1 medium red onion, peeled and cut into chunks
- Salt and pepper to taste

DIRECTIONS

1. In a shallow bowl stir together curry powder, yogurt, lemon juice and agave until smooth. Marinate chicken cubes in the curry mixture for at least 30 minutes.

2. Heat an outdoor or indoor grill to medium-high and coat lightly with oil. Thread skewers with chicken, bell pepper and onion and season with salt and pepper.

3. Grill kebabs on all sides until browned and chicken juices run clear, about 12 minutes. Serve immediately.

INFORMATION

Makes 2 servings
Calories: 206 per serving

SERVING TIP

Serve each portion with 1 cup white or brown basmati rice and a green salad tossed with light dressing for 480 calories.

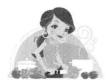 *" Buddy up with someone and exercise with them*

CHICKEN IN MUSHROOM SAUCE

Unbelievably rich and creamy, this dish is sure to satisfy any appetite for an extraordinary entrée that's quick to prepare.

INGREDIENTS

- 1 tsp. olive oil
- 2 boneless, skinless, chicken breasts, cut into 1-inch cubes
- Salt and pepper to taste
- 1 small onion, finely chopped
- 1 cup thinly sliced white mushrooms
- 1 tbsp. apple juice
- 1 cup low-sodium chicken broth or water
- ½ cup nonfat evaporated milk
- 2 tsp. prepared mustard
- 1 tsp. cornstarch

DIRECTIONS

1. Heat the oil in a large nonstick pan over medium-high heat. Season the chicken with salt and pepper and cook in the oil, stirring frequently to lightly brown, about 2 minutes. Transfer with a slotted spoon to a plate and set aside.

2. Add the onion and mushrooms to the skillet and cook, stirring often, until somewhat softened and lightly browned, about 4 minutes. Return the chicken with its juices to the pan and add the apple juice and broth. Stir well and cook for 1 minute over high heat. Cover, reduce the heat to low and cook until the chicken is firm and no longer pink inside, about 8 minutes.

3. In a small bowl whisk together the milk, mustard and cornstarch. Stir the mixture into the pan and bring to a simmer. Continue cooking for 2 minutes until the sauce is thick and rich. Taste for seasoning and serve immediately.

Information

Makes 2 servings
Calories: 228 per serving

Serving Tip

Serve each portion with ½ cup plain egg noodles, 1 cup steamed string beans and an apple for 488 calories.

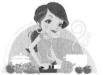

" Commit to making one positive change each day for your health and fitness

BAKED SHELLFISH PAELLA

This healthy version of a Spanish classic made with brown basmati rice is a snap to put together and will provide terrific leftovers for busy nights.

INGREDIENTS

- 1 tbsp. olive oil
- ½ medium onion, chopped
- ½ medium green bell pepper, seeded and diced
- Salt and pepper to taste
- 2 garlic cloves, minced
- ½ cup uncooked brown basmati rice
- 1 ½ cups low-sodium chicken or vegetable broth
- 1 ½ cup canned diced tomatoes, drained
- 1 bay leaf
- Pinch crushed saffron threads
- 1 lb. uncooked large shrimp, peeled and deveined
- 1 dozen clams, scrubbed
- 1 ½ dozen mussels in shell, scrubbed
- ¼ cup frozen green peas, thawed
- 1 tsp. finely chopped fresh parsley leaves
- Lemon wedges for serving

DIRECTIONS

1. Preheat the oven to 350 °F.

2. Heat the oil in a Dutch oven or other heavy-bottomed oven proof pot over medium-high heat. Add onion and bell pepper, season with salt and pepper and cook, stirring often, until somewhat softened, about 3 minutes. Add garlic and cook a further minute.

3. Add rice and stir to coat with onion mixture. Add broth, tomatoes, bay leaf and saffron and bring to a boil, stirring occasionally. Remove from heat, cover and transfer to the oven. Cook until most of the liquid is absorbed, about 35 minutes.

4. Remove from oven, stir and place shrimp, clams, mussels and green peas on top. Cover and return to oven and cook until rice is tender, shrimp is opaque and clam and mussel shells have opened, about 20 minutes.

5. Let stand, covered, for 5 minutes. Discard any unopened clams or mussels. Sprinkle with parsley and serve immediately with lemon wedges.

INFORMATION

Makes 4 servings
Calories: 292 per serving

SERVING TIP

Serve each portion with a large tossed salad lightly dressed and ½ cup plain yogurt with ½ cup berries and a drizzle of honey for 470 calories.

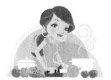

❝ *Steady weight loss is best -
don't try and rush things*

SWORDFISH STEAK WITH YOGURT PARSLEY SAUCE

Swordfish is great for the grill and easy to cook alongside assorted grilled veggies in this delicious and healthy recipe.

INGREDIENTS

- 1 4 oz. swordfish steak
- Juice of ½ lemon
- 1 tsp. olive oil
- Salt and pepper to taste
- Dash paprika

For the parsley sauce:

- 2 tbsp. nonfat plain Greek yogurt
- 1 tbsp. low-fat milk
- 1 ½ tbsp. finely chopped fresh parsley
- 1 tsp. capers, drained, rinsed and chopped

DIRECTIONS

1. Place the swordfish in a shallow baking dish in a single layer. Drizzle the lemon and oil over and season with the salt and pepper. Add a dash of paprika and marinate in the refrigerator for at least 1 hour.

2. Heat an outdoor or indoor grill to medium-high. Meanwhile, whisk together the sauce ingredients in a small bowl and refrigerate until ready to serve.

3. Grill the fish until firm and white and the edges begin to brown, about 6 minutes per side. Transfer to a serving dish and serve with the sauce on the side.

INSTRUCTIONS

Makes 1 serving
Calories: 207 per serving

SERVING TIP

Serve with 1½ cups assorted grilled vegetables such as zucchini, eggplant, bell peppers and onions and a wholegrain roll for 455 calories.

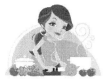

❝ *Try something new each week so that you are not bored by the food you eat*

CRISPY OVEN FRIED CHICKEN

This low-fat "fried" chicken recipe also boasts the terrific flavor of coconut.

INGREDIENTS

- 8 oz. boneless skinless chicken breasts
- ½ cup low-fat coconut milk
- Salt and pepper to taste
- 1 ¼ cups corn flakes, crushed
- ¼ cup unsweetened flaked coconut
- Drizzle of coconut oil, melted or canola oil

DIRECTIONS

1. Preheat the oven to 375 °F. Line a rimmed baking sheet with parchment paper.

2. Cut each breast in half and place in a glass or ceramic dish. Pour the coconut milk over. Allow to marinate at least 30 minutes.

3. In a shallow bowl, combine the salt, pepper, crushed corn flakes and flaked coconut. Dredge each chicken piece in the corn flake mixture, pressing firmly to adhere and place on the prepared baking sheet.

4. Drizzle the melted coconut oil over each and bake, turning once, until the chicken is cooked through and the crust begins to brown, about 30 minutes. Remove from the oven and allow to rest for 10 minutes before serving.

INFORMATION

Makes 2 servings
Calories: 265 per serving

SERVING TIP

Serve each portion with 2tbsp. of Duck sauce for dipping, ½ cup steamed spinach and ½ medium sweet potato for 478 calories.

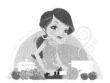

 Even a little extra exercise makes a huge difference

Boneless Pork Provence Style

Extremely lean pork fillets highlight this great low-fat cooking method that makes clean up a breeze.

Ingredients

- 4 oz. thin cut boneless pork fillets
- Salt and pepper to taste
- ¼ cup thinly sliced onion
- ½ cup thinly sliced red, orange, or green bell pepper
- 1 plum tomato, sliced
- Splash of white wine or apple juice
- Pinch dried Herbes de Provence

Directions

1. Preheat the oven to 350 °F. Place a rimmed baking sheet in the oven while heating.

2. Place a 12-in piece of foil on a flat surface and fan out the pork in the middle. Sprinkle with salt and pepper. Place the vegetables evenly on top, add the wine and herbs and close up the foil into an airtight tent shape.

3. Place on the heated baking sheet and cook for 20 to 25 minutes. You can carefully open the packet to check that the pork is no longer pink.

4. Open the packet on the baking sheet and briefly turn on the broiler just to lightly brown, for 1 or 2 minutes. Serve immediately.

INFORMATION

Makes 1 serving
Calories: 195 per serving

SERVING TIP

Serve each portion with 3 small boiled red-skin potatoes with light margarine and an apple for 475 calories.

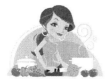

❝ *Cut down on alcohol
(or cut it out completely)*

CURRIED VEGETARIAN STEW

Exotic Indian flavor highlights this medley of nutritious vegetables and protein-rich beans for a terrific entrée that's low in calories and fat.

INGREDIENTS

- 1 tsp. canola oil
- ½ medium onion, chopped
- ½ medium red bell pepper, cored, seeded and diced
- Salt and pepper to taste
- 1 tbsp. minced fresh ginger
- 2 garlic cloves, minced
- ½ small jalapeno pepper, seeded and minced
- 1 tbsp. curry powder, mild or hot
- ½ tsp. ground turmeric
- ¼ tsp. ground coriander
- 1 cup vegetable broth or water
- ½ cup unsweetened low-fat coconut milk
- ¼ cup no-salt-added tomato sauce
- ¼ cup dried red lentils
- 1 medium sweet potato, peeled and cubed
- 1 cup shelled edamame beans
- 1 cup Indian paneer cheese (or tofu), cubed

DIRECTIONS

1. Heat the oil in a medium pot over medium-high heat. Add the onion, bell pepper, salt and pepper and cook, stirring often, until softened, about 3 minutes.

2. Add the ginger, garlic and jalapeno and cook, stirring, a further minute. Add the curry powder, turmeric and coriander and stir well to coat the vegetables.

3. Add the broth, coconut milk and tomato sauce and bring to a simmer. Add the lentils, sweet potatoes and edamame, reduce the heat to low, cover and simmer until the vegetables are tender, 12 to 15 minutes.

4. When the vegetables are tender, add the paneer and simmer until heated through. Taste for seasoning and serve immediately.

INFORMATION

Make 2 servings
Calories: 320 per serving

SERVING TIP

Serve each portion with 1 cup white or brown basmati rice and a dollop of plain yogurt for 495 calories.

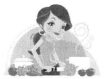

66 *Don't get hung up on your weight - aim for a healthy diet and lifestyle instead*

ITALIAN VEGETABLE BURRITOS

Italian flavors add variety to this quick vegetarian burrito recipe that's a delicious low-fat take on Mexican fare.

INGREDIENTS

- 1 tsp. olive oil
- ¼ medium red bell pepper, cored, seeded and sliced
- 1 small onion, halved and sliced
- 1 cup diced summer squash (zucchini and yellow)
- Salt and pepper to taste
- ¼ cup fava or lima beans, drained
- ½ cup diced extra-firm tofu
- 1 tbsp. chopped fresh basil
- 2 medium-size tortillas, warmed
- ½ cup low-fat shredded mozzarella cheese

DIRECTIONS

1. Heat olive oil in a nonstick skillet over medium high heat. Add bell pepper and onion and cook, stirring often, until slightly softened, about 3 minutes.

2. Add squash, salt and pepper and stir. Continue to cook until squash is just fork tender, about 2 minutes more. Add beans, tofu and basil, cover and cook for 2 minutes until heated through.

3. Spoon mixture onto heated tortillas, sprinkle with the cheese, fold up and serve.

INFORMATION

Makes 2 servings
Calories: 313 per serving

SERVING TIP

Serve with a large lightly dressed Italian salad for 425 calories.

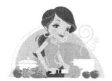

" *You can always revise or add new goals once you achieve the ones you have set*

GREEK STYLE MEATBALLS

Part meatball, part rice ball, you'll love these easy to make Greek favorites that are full of flavor and lean protein.

INGREDIENTS

For the meatballs

- 8 oz. ground lamb or beef
- Salt and pepper to taste
- ¼ cooked brown rice
- 2 tbsp. bread crumbs
- ½ small onion, finely chopped
- 3 sundried tomato pieces, finely chopped
- 1 tsp. each chopped fresh dill, mint and parsley
- 1 large egg white, slightly beaten

For the sauce:

- 2 tsp. olive oil
- 2/3 cup water
- Juice of ½ lemon
- 1 tsp. cornstarch

DIRECTIONS

1. In a medium bowl combine all the ingredients for the meatballs and mix well using your hands. Shape into walnut sized balls and place on a sheet of wax paper. Set aside.

2. Heat the olive oil in a large nonstick skillet over medium-high heat. Add the meatballs, one at a time, allowing a little space in between each. Cook over medium heat, turning occasionally to brown evenly.

3. Add the water to the skillet, stir and scrape up any browned bits, cover, reduce the heat to low and cook until the meatballs are firm and no longer pink inside, 5 to 8 minutes.

4. Remove the cover, stir together the lemon juice and cornstarch, add to the skillet and swirl the pan to create a light coating of a sauce for the meatballs. Serve immediately.

INFORMATION

Makes 2 servings
Calories: 218 per serving

SERVING TIP

Serve each portion with a small whole wheat pita, 2 tbsp. tzaziki yogurt sauce, a lightly dressed green salad and 1 cup grapes for 485 calories.

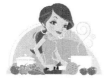

" *Sticking with a small change is much better than a large change you can't maintain*

PERFECT BEEF STEW

Hearty is the only way to describe this weeknight stew that's easy to make and wonderful to enjoy.

INGREDIENTS

- 1 tbsp. olive oil
- 1 lb. lean stewing beef, cubed and trimmed of excess fat
- Salt and pepper to taste
- 1 tsp. flour for dusting
- 1 medium onion, chopped
- 1 medium celery stalk, chopped
- 2 garlic cloves, minced
- 1 tbsp. tomato paste
- 2 tsp. no-sugar-added redcurrant jelly
- 2 cups low-sodium beef broth
- 1 ½ cups water
- 1 bay leaf
- 2 large carrots, peeled and cut into 1-inch chunks
- 2 medium turnips, peeled and quartered
- 1 cup diced butternut squash

DIRECTIONS

1. Heat oil in a large heavy-bottomed pot over medium-high heat. Season beef with salt and pepper, dust with flour and fry in the oil until browned on all sides, 5 to 7 minutes. Remove beef from pot and set aside.

2. Add onion and celery to pot and cook over medium heat, stirring often, until softened, about 4 minutes. Add garlic and cook a further minute.

3. Stir in tomato paste and jelly and continue to cook, stirring constantly, for 2 minutes. Add stock, water and bay leaf, increase heat to high and bring to a boil. Return beef to pot, reduce heat to medium-low and simmer, covered, until nearly fork tender, about 1 hour.

4. Add carrots and cook at a simmer for 10 minutes. Add turnips and squash and cook, stirring occasionally, until beef and vegetables are completely tender, 10 to 20 minutes. Add water if necessary, to prevent sticking and maintain gravy consistency. Serve immediately.

INFORMATION

Makes 4 servings
Calories: 362 per serving

SERVING TIP

Serve with a small wholegrain roll and a lightly dressed green bean salad for 498 calories.

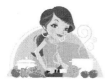 66 *Eat healthily to stay healthy for life*

Carrot, Sweet Potato and Ginger Bisque

You'll love the creamy consistency of this delightful fall soup that's great to enjoy any time of year.

Ingredients

- 1 tbsp. olive oil
- 1 medium leek (white part only), trimmed, washed well and chopped
- One 2-inch piece fresh ginger, peeled and chopped
- 6 cups low-sodium chicken or vegetable broth
- ½ tsp. ground cinnamon
- Dash ground nutmeg
- 1 lb carrots, trimmed peeled and sliced
- 2 medium sweet potatoes, peeled and cubed
- Salt and pepper to taste

Directions

1. In a heavy-bottomed soup pot, heat oil over medium heat, then add the leek and ginger and cook, stirring, until the leeks are soft and translucent, about 10 minutes. Do not brown.

2. Add the broth, cinnamon and nutmeg and stir well to combine. Add the carrots and sweet potatoes, bring to a simmer and allow to cook, uncovered, until the vegetables are fork tender, 25 to 30 minutes. Season with pepper.

3. Carefully transfer the hot soup in batches to a blender and process until smooth. Transfer to a clean pot or soup tureen. If the consistency is too thick, add a little more broth or water. Taste for salt and pepper, adjust as necessary and serve hot.

INFORMATION

Makes 4 servings
Calories: 220 per serving

SERVING TIP

Serve with a small lightly dressed chef's salad for 455 calories.

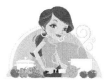

66 *There is no need to add sugar to your drinks – go without, you'll soon get used to it*

CURRIED LENTIL SOUP

A hint of curry is the magic ingredient in this delicious soup featuring the king of legumes - protein-rich lentils.

INGREDIENTS

- 1 tbsp. olive oil
- 1 medium onion, diced
- 1 medium celery stalk, diced
- 1 garlic clove, minced
- 1 pkg. (16 oz.) dried brown lentils, picked over and rinsed
- 6 cups low-sodium chicken or vegetable stock
- 1 tbsp. mild curry powder
- Salt and pepper to taste

DIRECTIONS

1. Heat oil in a soup pot over medium heat, add onion and celery and cook until softened, 8 to 10 minutes, stirring often. Stir in garlic and cook a further minute.

2. Stir in broth, lentils and curry powder, increase heat to high and bring to a boil. Reduce heat to medium-low and cook at a simmer, stirring occasionally, until lentils are soft but firm to the bite, about 25 minutes. Add water if necessary to thin.

3. Transfer 2 cups of soup to a blender and purée. Return to the pot, season with salt and pepper and serve immediately.

INFORMATION

Makes 6 servings
Calories: 220 per serving

SERVING TIP

Serve with a large tossed salad and a small roll for 368 calories.

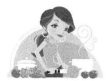

" *Be aware of the hidden calories in what you use to cook*

Fettuccine with Creamy Yogurt Sauce

Greek yogurt and cottage cheese provide the richness and protein in this amazing pasta dish that will become a real favorite.

Ingredients

- 4 to 6 oz. egg fettuccine or spaghetti
- Salt to taste
- 2 tsp. olive oil
- 1 medium shallot, finely chopped
- 1 cup nonfat plain Greek yogurt
- 1 1/3 cup low-fat whipped cottage cheese
- Freshly ground pepper
- 2 tsp. grated Parmesan cheese

Directions

1. Bring a pot of salted water to boil over high heat to cook the fettuccine.

2. Heat the oil in a medium nonstick saucepan over medium heat, add the shallot, sprinkle with salt and cook until softened, about 2 minutes, being careful not to brown. Whisk in the yogurt and cottage cheese, remove from the heat and set aside.

3. Cook the fettuccine according to the package directions. Transfer with tongs to the saucepan, adding a little of the pasta water to thin the sauce. Stir well to coat and add the freshly ground pepper. Taste for the addition of salt.

4. Serve immediately sprinkled with the cheese.

INFORMATION

Makes 2 servings
Calories: 260 per serving

SERVING TIP

Serve with a large tossed Italian salad for 375 calories.

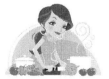

66 Visualize how you want to be, don't think about how you are right now

LENTIL SHEPHERD'S PIE

Hearty legumes and tempeh take the place of ground beef in this delicious casserole topped with mashed sweet potatoes.

INGREDIENTS

- 1 tsp. canola oil
- 1 medium onion, chopped
- 1 small celery stalk, chopped
- Salt and pepper to taste
- 1 tbsp. flour
- ½ tsp. dried thyme
- 2 (15 oz.) cans cooked lentils, drained
- ½ cup crumbled tempeh
- ¼ cup frozen peas, thawed
- 1 cup vegetable broth or water
- 2 medium sweet potatoes, peeled and diced
- ¼ cup lowfat milk
- Dash ground cinnamon

DIRECTIONS

1. Heat oil in a large nonstick skillet over medium-high heat. Add onion and celery and season with salt and pepper. Cook stirring occasionally, until softened, about 6 minutes.

2. Stir in flour and cook for 1 minute. Add thyme, lentils, tempeh, peas and broth and continue cooking, stirring often, until broth has thickened and vegetables are heated through, about 5 minutes. Set aside.

3. Preheat the oven to 350 °F. Lightly grease a 9 x 9-inch baking dish.

4. In a medium saucepan, place sweet potatoes, a good pinch of salt and water to cover. Bring to a boil, reduce heat to a simmer and cook until fork tender, about 10 minutes. Drain well and set aside.

5. Transfer lentil mixture to casserole and spread evenly. Place potatoes in a medium bowl with milk and cinnamon and mash to desired consistency. Season with salt and pepper and spread on top of lentil mixture, smoothing decoratively with the tines of a fork.

6. Bake until edges of pie begin to bubble and lentil mixture is piping hot, 30 to 40 minutes. Serve immediately.

INFORMATION

Makes 4 servings
Calories: 325

SERVING TIP

Serve with a tossed green salad for 415 calories.

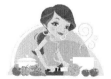

“ *Several small positive changes can combine to make a huge change*

Turkey Paprikas

Enjoy this traditional Hungarian dish made healthy and creamy with the addition of Greek yogurt.

Ingredients

- 1 tsp. olive oil
- ½ medium onion, chopped
- Salt and pepper taste
- 1 garlic clove, minced
- 8 oz. cooked turkey breast, shredded
- 2 tsp. paprika
- 1 cup low sodium chicken broth
- ¼ cup nonfat plain Greek yogurt

Directions

1. Heat oil in a nonstick skillet over medium-high heat. Add onion, season with salt and pepper and cook until softened, about 4 minutes. Add garlic and cook a further minute.

2. Stir in turkey and sprinkle with paprika. Stir well to combine.

3. Pour in chicken broth and bring to a simmer. Stir in yogurt and continue to cook over very low heat until thickened and well heated through.

4. Taste for additional seasoning and serve immediately.

INFORMATION

Makes 2 servings
Calories: 249 per serving

SERVING TIP

Serve with 1 cup lightly buttered egg noodles and a tossed green salad for 440 calories.

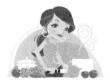

“ *A healthy diet will help reduce and prevent obesity, as well as obesity-related problems such as infertility, heart disease and cancer*

Terrific Turkey Loaf

Deliciously moist with a hint of aromatic herbs, this healthy loaf will quickly become a dinner time favorite.

Ingredients

- 1 lb ground turkey
- 1 small onion, finely chopped
- 1 garlic clove, minced
- Salt and pepper to taste
- 2 tsp. dried parsley
- 1 tsp. dried marjoram
- 1 tsp. dried thyme
- 1 large egg, beaten
- ½ cup unseasoned bread crumbs

Directions

1. Preheat the oven to 325 °F.

2. In a medium mixing bowl combine all the ingredients and mix well.

3. Transfer to a glass or ceramic 8 x 3-inch loaf pan and pat down to remove any air pockets.

4. Cover tightly with foil and bake until an instant read thermometer inserted in the middle reaches 165 °F, 35 to 45 minutes. Remove foil during the final 10 minutes to brown.

5. Allow to rest for 10 minutes before slicing and serving.

INFORMATION

Makes 4 servings
Calories: 285 per serving

SERVING TIP

Serve each portion with ½ cup whole grain couscous or pasta, 1 cup steamed green beans and 1 cup strawberries for 495 calories.

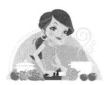 **❝** *Why not grow your own herbs?*

BUFFALO CHICKEN BITES

No need to give up the great taste of Buffalo wings with this easy and healthy rendition.

INGREDIENTS

- 8 oz. boneless skinless chicken breasts
- Salt and pepper to taste
- ½ cup hot sauce such as Frank's
- 1 large egg white, beaten
- 1 cup panko breadcrumbs
- 1 tsp. garlic powder
- 1 tsp. paprika
- 2 tsp. light butter, melted
- Reduced fat blue cheese dressing
- Celery sticks

DIRECTIONS

1. Preheat the oven to 400 °F. Line a baking sheet with parchment paper.

2. Cut the chicken into bite-size pieces, season with salt and pepper and set aside.

3. In a small bowl combine hot sauce and egg white. In another bowl combine breadcrumbs, garlic powder and paprika.

4. Dip chicken pieces into hot sauce mixture then dredge in breadcrumb mixture and place on prepared baking sheet. Drizzle with the melted butter and bake until crispy and browned, turning once, 8 to 12 minutes. Serve with the dressing and celery.

INFORMATION

Makes 2 servings
Calories: 317 per serving

SERVING TIP

Serve with a large tossed salad and crispy Idaho oven fries for 490 calories.

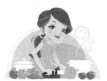

" Plan ahead for meals so that you have the items you'll need

DARK CHOCOLATE PUDDING

You'll relish every spoonful of this rich and delicious dessert with its intense chocolate flavor and creamy consistency.

INGREDIENTS

- 1 ½ cups low-fat milk
- 1 large egg, beaten
- 1 tsp. vanilla
- 2 tbsp. cornstarch
- ¼ cup unsweetened cocoa powder
- ½ cup granulated sugar
- Pinch of salt
- 2 tbsp. chopped dark chocolate

DIRECTIONS

1. Combine milk, egg and vanilla in a medium saucepan.

2. Whisk together cornstarch, cocoa powder, sugar and salt in a small bowl.

3. Add cornstarch mixture to milk mixture in saucepan and whisking often, over medium heat, bring to a simmer and cook, lightly bubbling, for 2 to 3 minutes, or until thickened. Switch to a wooden spoon for stirring as mixture becomes thicker.

4. Remove from heat and stir in dark chocolate.

5. Transfer to dessert cups and refrigerate for at least 1 hour before serving.

INFORMATION

Makes 4 servings
Calories: 189 per serving

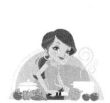

" *Treat yourself with non-food items, such as a bath or a book*

APPLE CRUMB PIES

INGREDIENTS

- ½ tsp. light butter
- 2 Granny Smith apples, peeled, cored, and cut into ¼-inch thick slices
- ½ cup unsweetened applesauce
- 1/8 tsp. ground cinnamon
- 1 tsp. honey
- 1 tsp. lemon juice

For the topping:

¼ cup flour
1 tbsp. light butter
2 tsp. light brown sugar
Dash ground cinnamon

DIRECTIONS

1. Preheat the oven to 350 degrees F. Lightly brush 2 medium-size ramekins or custard cups with the butter.

2. In a medium bowl combine the apples with the remaining ingredients, except those for the topping and stir well. Spoon into each ramekin evenly. In a small bowl combine topping ingredients until the mixture resembles sand and sprinkle over each apple pie.

3. Transfer the 2 dishes to a baking sheet and bake until the apples are soft and the topping is golden, 20 to 30 minutes. Serve while still warm.

INFORMATION

Makes 2 servings
Calories: 168 per serving

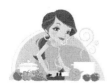

" *Get to know your own body and your level of hunger*

INCREDIBLE CARAMEL CUSTARD

Traditionally made with caramelized sugar, this flavorful and rich dessert gets a low carb makeover with the help of sweetener, agave and the intoxicating aroma of vanilla bean.

INGREDIENTS

- 1 cup milk
- 1 2-inch piece vanilla bean, unopened
- 2 packets sugar substitute
- 2 tsp. sugar-free caramel syrup
- 5 large egg yolks, beaten
- Amber agave nectar or honey, for serving

DIRECTIONS

1. Heat milk with vanilla bean in a small saucepan over medium heat until just warmed. Set aside for 10 minutes.

2. Preheat the oven to 325 °F. Line a small 3-inch tall roasting pan with parchment paper. Lightly coat 4 half cup ramekins or ovenproof dessert cups with cooking spray.

3. In a medium bowl whisk together sugar substitute, caramel syrup and egg yolks until well combined.

4. Remove vanilla bean from milk and slowly pour into egg mixture, whisking well. Divide mixture between prepared ramekins and place in roasting pan.

5. Pour boiling water into roasting pan to come halfway up sides of ramekins and carefully place entire pan into the oven.

6. Bake for 30 to 40 minutes or until the custard is set and a toothpick comes out clean.

7. Remove from oven and carefully lift ramekins of pan, placing on a flat plate or tray. Refrigerate until completely cooled.

8. To serve, run a sharp paring knife around the edge of the ramekin and turn out onto a dessert plate. Drizzle with agave and serve.

INFORMATION

Makes 4 servings
Calories: 140 per serving

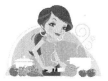

66 *You can judge your weight by the way your clothing feels on you, not just by the scales*

Weights

½ oz	10g
¾ oz	20g
1 oz	25g
1½ oz	40g
2 oz	50g
2½ oz	60g
3 oz	75g
4 oz	110g
4½ oz	125g
5 oz	150g
6 oz	175g
7 oz	200g
8 oz	225g
9 oz	250g
10 oz	275g
12 oz	350g
1 lb	450g
2 lb	900g
3 lb	1350g

Liquid Measures

1 tbsp	½ fl. oz	15ml
1/8 cup	1fl.oz	30ml
¼ cup	2fl.oz	60ml
½ cup	4fl.oz	120ml
1 cup	8fl.oz	240ml
1 pint	16fl.oz	480ml

Temperatures

°F	°C	Gas Mark
275°F	140°C	1
300°F	150°C	2
325°F	170°C	3
350°F	180°C	4
375°F	190°C	5
400°F	200°C	6
425°F	210°C	7
450°F	220°C	8
475°F	230°C	9

American Cup Measures

1 cup flour	5oz	150g
1 cup caster/ granulated sugar	8oz	225g
1 cup brown sugar	6oz	175g
1 cup butter/margarine/lard	8oz	225g
1 cup sultanas/raisins	7oz	200g
1 cup currants	5oz	150g
1 cup ground almonds	4oz	110g
1 cup golden syrup	12oz	350g
1 cup uncooked rice	7oz	200g
1 cup grated cheese	4oz	110g
1 stick butter	4oz	110g

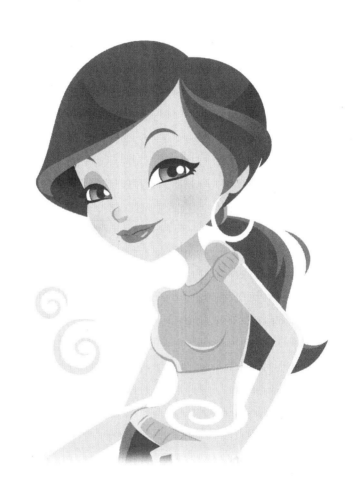

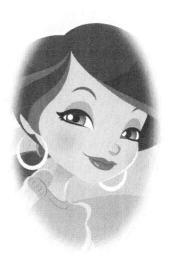

AUTHOR BIO

Beth Christian is not a doctor or nutritionist, she's a busy mom who needs to keep fit and healthy. She loves her food and wants to help others overcome their love-hate relationship with it, and enjoy a long, healthy life.

100 Under 500 Calorie Meals

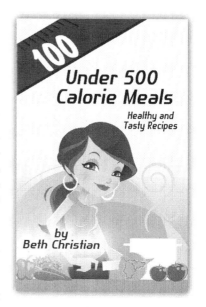

The perfect collection of 100 easy-to-make, nutrient-rich, delicious, calorie-counted recipes which can be mixed and matched to give you a satisfying meal of 500 calories or less.

Written to be used by anyone embarking on a weight-loss plan, calorie-counted diet or those just looking to eat more healthily.

Each recipe is calorie-counted, so it is easy to keep track of calories and to combine recipes for the perfect main meal. The main meal recipes also include tips on what sides to serve them with and how many calories these add. If you want a lighter lunch then simply combine a salad and soup, or a salad and dessert. Those with a sweet tooth will enjoy the nice (but not naughty!) desserts of 200 calories or less.

This book will support you with your weight loss goals and help you follow a healthy eating plan without compromising on taste and variety.

100 **Under 500 Calorie Meals** includes hearty soups, salads, main meals, poultry, fish and shellfish, meat and vegetarian, sides, 200 calorie (or less) desserts and reduced calorie Holiday menus.

> **BONUS:** Contains tips written by Beth to help
> you really achieve the healthy life you want.

Other Books from MadeGlobal Publishing

Please Leave a Review

If you enjoyed this book, please leave a review on Amazon or at the book seller where you purchased it. There is no better way to thank the author and it really does make a huge difference! Thank you in advance.

Visit the Website for the Book:

http://easyalternatedayfasting.com/

You'll find tips, ideas and more things to help you achieve the life you want. We look forward to seeing you there.

Made in the USA
Lexington, KY
30 March 2013